AI Longevity After 40

How Artificial Intelligence Identifies Early Aging Signals and Protects Your Health Before Decline Begins

By Joe Correa

Published by Live Stronger Faster

This book is for educational and informational purposes only. The author and publisher are not engaged in rendering legal, financial, or other professional advice. Readers should consult a qualified professional before making any financial decisions.

First Edition

Table of Contents

Introduction

Turning forty is not a crisis, but it is a biological checkpoint. Long before symptoms appear, long before a doctor raises a concern, and long before most people realize anything has changed, the body begins to shift its internal priorities. Cellular repair slows slightly. Hormonal signaling becomes less efficient. Muscle protein synthesis begins to decline. Inflammation becomes easier to trigger and harder to resolve. These changes are not dramatic, and that is precisely why they are so dangerous. Aging after forty rarely announces itself loudly. It works quietly, subtly, and cumulatively, laying the groundwork for fatigue, metabolic dysfunction, joint pain, cognitive fog, cardiovascular stress, and chronic disease years or even decades later. The purpose of this book is to explain why aging accelerates after forty, how artificial intelligence can detect the earliest signals of decline before symptoms appear, and how you can use AI-powered insights to protect your health long before damage becomes irreversible.

For decades, healthcare has been reactive. Most people are told they are healthy until a lab result crosses a predefined threshold, an image reveals structural damage, or symptoms interfere with daily life. By the time traditional medicine intervenes, biological decline has already been underway for years. Artificial intelligence changes this model entirely. Instead of waiting for disease to appear, AI analyzes patterns across thousands or millions of variables, identifying deviations from your personal baseline long before they meet diagnostic criteria. This shift—from reactive medicine to predictive health—is especially powerful after forty, when the difference between early intervention and delayed response can mean decades of preserved vitality or decades of unnecessary decline.

This book is not about chasing youth, denying age, or adopting extreme longevity experiments. It is about understanding how aging actually works after forty and using intelligent systems to slow, stabilize, and optimize the process. Aging is not a single process; it is the cumulative result of multiple systems drifting out of balance. These systems include metabolic regulation, immune response, hormonal signaling, musculoskeletal integrity, cardiovascular efficiency, mitochondrial energy production, and neural communication. Artificial intelligence excels at analyzing systems, not just isolated data points. That is why AI is uniquely suited to longevity science, especially for adults entering midlife.

After forty, the most critical threat to long-term health is not a specific disease but silent acceleration. Small inefficiencies compound. Slight insulin resistance becomes metabolic syndrome. Minor muscle loss becomes frailty. Subclinical inflammation becomes cardiovascular disease. AI identifies these trajectories early by recognizing patterns invisible to human interpretation. It compares your biomarkers, activity data, sleep cycles, stress responses, nutritional inputs, and genetic predispositions against massive datasets to detect where aging is beginning to speed up. The earlier these patterns are identified, the easier they are to correct.

One of the most important concepts you will learn in this book is that chronological age and biological age are not the same. Two people can be forty-five years old on paper and differ biologically by twenty years. Artificial intelligence allows biological age to be estimated with increasing precision by integrating blood markers, imaging data, movement patterns, and lifestyle inputs. This matters because the goal of longevity is not to add years at the end of life but to protect function, strength, clarity, and independence throughout life. AI does not guess. It measures trends, predicts outcomes, and models interventions with unprecedented accuracy.

Many people assume that aging after forty is inevitable and linear, but this belief is outdated. Aging accelerates when systems fall out of coordination. AI identifies where coordination is failing. For example, slight disruptions in circadian rhythm can cascade into hormonal imbalance, insulin dysregulation, poor sleep quality, increased inflammation, and cognitive decline. AI systems track these interconnections continuously, allowing targeted interventions before damage becomes entrenched. This is not theoretical. These tools are already being used in advanced preventive medicine, performance optimization, and longevity clinics worldwide.

This book is designed to translate complex AI-driven longevity science into clear, practical understanding. You will not need a technical background to benefit from these insights. Each concept is explained in plain language, with an emphasis on how AI tools work, what they measure, and how their findings apply to real life after forty. You will learn how AI analyzes blood panels differently than traditional medicine, how wearable data becomes predictive rather than descriptive, and how machine learning models identify risk patterns years ahead of symptoms.

Importantly, this book also addresses fear and misinformation. Artificial intelligence is often portrayed as cold, invasive, or dehumanizing. In reality, when used responsibly, AI restores personalization to healthcare. It moves away from one-size-fits-all recommendations and toward precision guidance based on your unique biology. After forty, individuality matters more than ever. What worked in your twenties may no longer work, and what works for others may actively harm you. AI excels at personalization because it adapts continuously as your body changes.

The focus of this first book in the series is early detection and protection. You will learn how AI identifies subtle aging signals in metabolism, inflammation, muscle retention, cardiovascular efficiency, cognitive processing speed, and recovery capacity. These signals often appear years before clinical diagnosis. By understanding them now, you gain leverage. You gain time. And in longevity, time is the most valuable asset of all.

This introduction also sets the foundation for the books that follow. While this volume focuses on aging after forty, each subsequent book in the series addresses a specific phase or system of aging with increasing depth. Aging after fifty introduces different challenges than aging after forty. Aging after sixty introduces new priorities entirely. Muscle preservation, bone integrity, heart health, balance, disease prevention, and energy restoration each deserve focused attention. Artificial intelligence connects them all, creating a unified framework for intelligent aging.

Another critical theme you will encounter throughout this book is prevention without obsession. Longevity does not require perfection. It requires awareness, consistency, and intelligent feedback loops. AI provides feedback loops that were previously unavailable. Instead of guessing whether a change is working, AI measures the impact over time. Instead of reacting emotionally to short-term fluctuations, AI tracks long-term trends. This perspective reduces anxiety while increasing control, especially for adults navigating midlife transitions.

The role of technology in aging raises ethical questions, and this book addresses them honestly. AI is a tool, not a replacement for human judgment or medical care. The goal is not dependency but empowerment. When you understand how AI systems evaluate health, you become a better decision-maker. You ask better questions. You intervene earlier. You collaborate more effectively with healthcare providers. After forty, this collaboration becomes increasingly important as the margin for error narrows.

This book also reframes aging as an optimization problem rather than a decline narrative. Optimization does not mean maximizing everything at once. It means stabilizing key systems, reducing unnecessary stressors, and preserving capacity where it matters most. AI models excel at optimization because they evaluate trade-offs realistically. They recognize that improving one metric at the expense of another may accelerate aging overall. This systems-based thinking is essential for sustainable longevity. As you move through this book, you will begin to see aging differently. You will understand that decline is not sudden but cumulative, not inevitable but conditional. Artificial intelligence gives us the ability to see those conditions clearly for the first time. After forty, clarity is power. The sooner you gain it, the longer you can use it to protect your health, independence, and quality of life.

This introduction marks the beginning of a new framework for aging—one grounded in data, guided by intelligence, and centered on prevention rather than repair. The chapters that follow will explore the specific biological signals AI detects after forty, the tools that make this detection possible, and the practical implications for daily life. By the end of this book, you will not only understand how AI identifies early aging signals but how those insights can be used to protect your health long before decline begins.

Chapter 1

The Silent Acceleration of Aging After 40 and How AI Sees It First

Aging after forty does not begin with pain, diagnosis, or visible decline. It begins with small shifts in biological efficiency that most people never notice because they occur beneath conscious awareness. Cells become slightly less responsive to repair signals. Hormonal messaging becomes less precise. Recovery from stress, exercise, and poor sleep takes marginally longer. These changes are not dramatic enough to disrupt daily life, which is why they are often ignored. Yet they mark the beginning of accelerated biological aging. Artificial intelligence is uniquely capable of detecting this phase because it does not rely on symptoms. It relies on patterns, trajectories, and deviations from your personal baseline.

The human body is a system of systems, and aging is the gradual loss of coordination between them. After forty, this coordination begins to weaken in subtle ways. Blood sugar regulation may still fall within normal laboratory ranges, yet show increased variability. Inflammation markers may remain below diagnostic thresholds while trending upward year after year. Muscle mass may decline slowly even as body weight remains unchanged. AI identifies these changes not as isolated data points but as early indicators of systemic drift. This distinction is critical because traditional medicine is designed to identify disease, not drift. AI is designed to detect drift before it becomes disease.

One of the most significant changes after forty is the widening gap between perceived health and biological reality. Many people feel fine while underlying systems are under increasing strain. Artificial intelligence closes this gap by continuously analyzing longitudinal data rather than relying on snapshots in time. A single blood test may appear normal, but AI evaluates trends across months and years. It recognizes when recovery capacity is diminishing, when metabolic flexibility is narrowing, and when stress responses are becoming exaggerated. These are early aging signals that humans cannot reliably interpret without computational assistance.

Aging acceleration is driven largely by feedback loops. Small inefficiencies create compensatory responses that increase long-term stress. For example, slight insulin resistance leads to higher insulin output, which increases inflammation, which disrupts sleep, which further worsens insulin sensitivity. AI identifies these loops early by modeling interactions across systems. It does not ask whether a value is normal. It asks whether a pattern is sustainable. After forty, sustainability becomes more important than optimization. AI excels at distinguishing between short-term performance and long-term resilience.

Another key aging signal after forty is the decline in adaptive capacity. Younger bodies adapt quickly to stressors such as intense exercise, poor sleep, or dietary changes. After forty, adaptation slows. AI detects this through changes in heart rate variability, recovery curves, cortisol rhythms, and sleep architecture. These metrics reveal whether the body is becoming more brittle or more resilient. Brittleness is the hallmark of accelerated aging. Resilience is the foundation of longevity. AI measures resilience continuously, offering early warnings when it begins to erode.

Inflammation deserves special attention because it is one of the earliest and most influential drivers of aging after forty. Chronic low-grade inflammation rarely causes immediate symptoms, yet it accelerates nearly every aging pathway. AI detects inflammatory drift by analyzing subtle changes in biomarkers, sleep quality, resting heart rate, and activity tolerance. It recognizes when the immune system is shifting from adaptive to reactive mode. This shift precedes cardiovascular disease, neurodegeneration, metabolic dysfunction, and musculoskeletal decline. Early detection allows for course correction before damage accumulates. Muscle loss also begins earlier than most people expect. After forty, muscle protein synthesis declines unless actively supported. The scale may not change, but body composition does. AI detects this through movement patterns, strength output, recovery time, and metabolic markers. It understands that muscle is not merely a structural tissue but a metabolic and endocrine organ. Loss of muscle accelerates aging across multiple systems. Identifying early muscle decline allows for targeted interventions that preserve strength and independence decades later.

Cognitive aging follows a similar pattern. After forty, processing speed, working memory, and cognitive flexibility may begin to decline subtly. AI detects this not through subjective complaints but through performance variability, reaction time, sleep-brain synchronization, and stress responses. These early changes are reversible when addressed promptly. Delayed intervention allows them to compound. AI shifts cognitive aging from an inevitable decline narrative to a manageable optimization challenge.

The most powerful advantage of AI in longevity science is personalization. Aging does not follow a universal timeline. Genetics, environment, stress exposure, nutrition, movement, and sleep interact uniquely for each individual. AI models adapt continuously, refining predictions as new data becomes available. This allows for early detection tailored to the individual rather than population averages. After forty, averages are misleading. Personalized trajectories are what matter.

Importantly, AI does not replace human judgment or medical care. It enhances them. By identifying early aging signals, AI allows individuals and clinicians to act proactively rather than reactively. This proactive stance reduces fear, increases clarity, and preserves agency. Aging becomes something to manage intelligently rather than endure passively. This shift in mindset is foundational for longevity after forty.

By understanding how aging accelerates silently and how AI detects it early, you gain the ability to intervene while change is still easy. The remainder of this book builds upon this foundation, exploring specific systems and tools that translate detection into protection. The earlier you engage with this process, the greater the return. Aging does not wait for awareness. Intelligence shortens the gap between change and response.

The Year Nothing Was "Wrong"

Daniel turned forty-three feeling healthy by every conventional standard. He exercised a few times a week, maintained a stable weight, and had no diagnosed conditions. His annual physical came back normal, and his doctor reassured him that he was doing well for his age. Yet something felt slightly off. Not enough to worry him, but enough to register quietly in the background. He took longer to recover from workouts. His sleep was lighter than it used to be. He felt mentally sharp most days but noticed occasional lapses in focus under stress. None of it seemed serious, so he ignored it.

At the suggestion of a colleague, Daniel began using an AI-powered health monitoring platform that integrated wearable data, blood work, and lifestyle inputs. He expected confirmation that everything was fine. Instead, the system revealed patterns he had never seen. His heart rate variability had been declining steadily for two years. His overnight glucose levels were increasingly volatile despite normal fasting labs. His sleep cycles showed reduced deep sleep after stressful days. Individually, none of these metrics were alarming. Together, they painted a picture of declining resilience.

The AI did not diagnose disease. It identified acceleration. It showed Daniel that his biological age was advancing faster than his chronological age, not because of a single issue but because of compounded stress and insufficient recovery. The system highlighted feedback loops he had never considered. Late workouts combined with evening screen exposure were disrupting sleep. Poor sleep was amplifying inflammation. Inflammation was slowing recovery. The loop was subtle but consistent. With guidance from the AI insights, Daniel made small, targeted changes. He shifted intense workouts earlier in the day. He adjusted protein intake to support muscle repair. He improved sleep timing and reduced late-night cognitive stimulation. None of these changes felt dramatic. Yet over the next six months, the AI tracked improvements in recovery curves, sleep depth, and metabolic stability. His biological age trajectory slowed.

What surprised Daniel most was how little he had felt before the changes. There had been no pain, no crisis, no diagnosis. The year nothing was "wrong" had been the year aging accelerated quietly. Without AI, he would have continued unaware until symptoms forced action. Instead, he intervened early, when change was easy and outcomes were reversible.

By the time Daniel turned forty-five, his metrics reflected restored resilience. He felt stronger, slept deeper, and handled stress more effectively. His doctor still saw normal labs, but Daniel understood something deeper. Longevity is not about waiting for decline. It is about recognizing drift. Artificial intelligence had given him visibility into a process that would otherwise have remained invisible. That visibility changed everything.

Chapter 2

How AI Measures Biological Age Instead of Calendar Age

Chronological age is a poor predictor of health, resilience, and longevity after forty. Two people born in the same year can differ dramatically in strength, cognitive clarity, metabolic health, and disease risk. What matters is not how many years you have lived, but how efficiently your biological systems are functioning. Artificial intelligence allows this distinction to be measured with increasing accuracy by shifting the focus from static markers to dynamic systems. Biological age reflects how well your body is aging internally, and after forty, this internal age becomes the most meaningful indicator of future health.

Traditional healthcare relies heavily on thresholds. Blood markers are labeled normal or abnormal based on population averages. Imaging results are classified as healthy or pathological. This binary framework obscures gradual decline because aging is not binary. It is progressive. AI replaces thresholds with trajectories. It evaluates how biomarkers change over time, how systems respond to stress, and how quickly the body returns to baseline. These patterns reveal biological age far more accurately than isolated measurements. Biological age is not a single number but a composite model.

AI integrates data from multiple domains including metabolic health, inflammation, cardiovascular function, musculoskeletal integrity, neurological performance, sleep architecture, and stress regulation. Each domain ages at a different rate. Some systems may remain youthful while others decline rapidly. AI identifies these imbalances, showing where aging is accelerating and where resilience remains strong. This systems-based view allows for targeted intervention rather than generalized recommendations.

One of the most important components of biological aging after forty is metabolic flexibility. The ability to efficiently switch between fuel sources, regulate blood glucose, and maintain insulin sensitivity declines subtly with age. AI detects this decline by analyzing glucose variability, post-meal responses, overnight metabolic stability, and energy patterns. These insights reveal metabolic aging years before diabetes or metabolic syndrome develops. Preserving metabolic flexibility slows aging across nearly every biological system.

Inflammatory burden is another major determinant of biological age. Chronic low-grade inflammation accelerates cellular damage, impairs repair mechanisms, and disrupts signaling pathways. AI measures inflammation indirectly as well as directly. Beyond blood markers, it analyzes sleep quality, resting heart rate trends, recovery time, and stress responses. This multidimensional approach reveals inflammatory aging even when traditional markers appear normal.

Musculoskeletal aging contributes significantly to biological age, particularly after forty. Muscle mass, strength output, coordination, and recovery capacity decline unless actively supported. AI evaluates movement efficiency, force production, fatigue patterns, and adaptation to training stimuli. It identifies early muscle aging that may not yet be visible through weight or appearance. Preserving muscle is one of the most effective ways to reduce biological age and extend healthspan.

Cardiovascular aging also progresses quietly. Arterial stiffness, autonomic imbalance, and reduced cardiovascular efficiency often develop without symptoms. AI detects these changes through heart rate variability, resting heart rate trends, blood pressure patterns, and exercise recovery. These metrics provide insight into vascular aging and autonomic nervous system health. Early detection allows for interventions that maintain cardiovascular youthfulness far beyond midlife.

Cognitive and neurological aging contribute heavily to perceived age and functional independence. AI measures cognitive aging through performance consistency, reaction time variability, sleep-brain synchronization, and stress-related cognitive decline. These indicators often change years before subjective cognitive complaints arise. Addressing them early preserves clarity, focus, and emotional regulation.

Sleep is a central regulator of biological age. After forty, sleep architecture often changes in subtle but meaningful ways. Deep sleep may decrease, REM cycles may fragment, and circadian rhythms may shift. AI analyzes sleep stages, timing consistency, and recovery impact. Poor sleep accelerates aging across all systems. AI does not simply label sleep as good or bad; it identifies how sleep quality influences biological aging trajectories.

What makes AI uniquely powerful is its ability to model interactions. Biological age accelerates when multiple systems decline together. AI identifies when metabolic stress amplifies inflammation, when poor sleep worsens cognitive aging, and when muscle loss reduces metabolic resilience. These interactions are invisible without computational modeling. Understanding them allows for precise, efficient interventions rather than scattered lifestyle changes.

Biological age is not fixed. AI models update continuously as inputs change. When interventions improve system function, biological age slows or even reverses. This feedback creates motivation grounded in evidence rather than hope. After forty, progress must be measurable to be sustainable. AI provides that measurement.

By shifting focus from chronological age to biological age, AI reframes aging as a dynamic process rather than an inevitable decline. This perspective empowers individuals to act early, prioritize intelligently, and preserve function long before symptoms appear. The rest of this book builds upon this foundation, translating biological age insights into practical longevity strategies.

Younger on Paper, Older Inside

Maria had just turned forty-six and felt proud of how well she was aging. Friends often commented that she looked younger than her age. She stayed active, maintained a healthy weight, and had no major medical issues. When her doctor told her she was "doing great for forty-six," she believed it completely. Yet she couldn't ignore a persistent sense of fatigue and mental fog that seemed to be creeping into her life.

At the encouragement of her daughter, Maria began using an AI-based biological age assessment that combined wearable data, blood markers, sleep analysis, and lifestyle tracking. She expected reassurance. Instead, the results startled her. Her chronological age was forty-six, but her biological age was estimated closer to fifty-four. The AI highlighted specific contributors: elevated inflammatory patterns, declining sleep efficiency, and reduced metabolic flexibility.

What unsettled Maria was not the number itself but the explanation. The AI showed her how each system interacted. Late meals disrupted sleep. Poor sleep increased inflammation. Inflammation impaired recovery and energy. The cycle repeated daily, gradually accelerating her biological aging. None of this had triggered a diagnosis. All of it was measurable.

With guided insights, Maria made focused adjustments rather than drastic changes. She improved sleep timing, adjusted meal composition, incorporated resistance training to preserve muscle, and reduced chronic stress exposure. The AI tracked changes monthly. Over the course of a year, her biological age estimate began to decline. At forty-seven, it measured closer to forty-three.

The changes were not just numerical. Maria felt sharper, more energetic, and more emotionally stable. Her doctor still saw normal labs, but Maria understood something deeper. Looking young meant nothing if systems were aging rapidly. Biological age told the truth her calendar never could.

By learning to measure aging correctly, Maria reclaimed control over her future health. AI had not frightened her. It had informed her. And that information became the foundation of lasting change.

Chapter 3

How AI Detects Early System Breakdown Before Symptoms Appear

Most people assume health problems begin when symptoms show up. In reality, symptoms are late-stage signals. By the time pain, fatigue, weakness, or cognitive issues appear, biological systems have already been under strain for years. After forty, the most dangerous phase of aging is not illness but invisible breakdown. Artificial intelligence is uniquely capable of detecting this breakdown because it does not wait for failure. It identifies weakening coordination between systems long before they collapse.

The human body functions as a network, not a collection of independent parts. Metabolism influences inflammation. Inflammation affects sleep. Sleep governs hormonal balance. Hormones regulate muscle, energy, mood, and cognition. When one system drifts out of alignment, others compensate. These compensations keep you functional but increase long-term stress. AI is designed to recognize compensation patterns. It sees when the body is working harder to maintain normal outcomes, which is the earliest warning sign of accelerated aging. One of the first breakdowns AI detects after forty is declining recovery efficiency. Recovery is not just rest;

it is the body's ability to return to baseline after stress. AI measures this through heart rate variability, sleep rebound patterns, post-exercise fatigue curves, and stress hormone rhythms. A younger system rebounds quickly. An aging system rebounds slowly and incompletely. This slowdown is rarely noticeable subjectively but is highly predictive of future decline. AI identifies this change years before people describe feeling "older."

Another early breakdown occurs in metabolic signaling. After forty, cells often respond less efficiently to insulin, cortisol, and growth signals. Blood tests may remain normal, yet variability increases. AI analyzes glucose fluctuations, energy dips, and stress responses across time. It identifies when metabolic regulation becomes unstable, even if average values appear healthy. Instability, not averages, is what drives aging acceleration.

Neurological system breakdown is also detected early by AI. Cognitive decline does not begin with memory loss. It begins with inconsistency. Reaction times vary more. Focus degrades under stress. Emotional regulation becomes less stable during fatigue. AI identifies these changes through performance variability, sleep-brain synchronization, and autonomic nervous system patterns. These signals appear long before clinical cognitive impairment and are often reversible when addressed early. Musculoskeletal breakdown is another silent process. Muscle loss, joint instability, and connective tissue weakening begin gradually after forty. AI evaluates movement efficiency, asymmetry, fatigue accumulation, and recovery from load. It recognizes when the body is compensating for weakness by altering movement patterns. These compensations increase injury risk and accelerate aging. Detecting them early allows for targeted strengthening before damage occurs.

Cardiovascular system breakdown is especially dangerous because it progresses quietly. Arterial stiffness, autonomic imbalance, and reduced vascular responsiveness often develop without symptoms. AI detects these changes through heart rate trends, variability patterns, blood pressure dynamics, and exercise recovery metrics. It recognizes when the cardiovascular system is losing adaptability, which is a strong predictor of future disease even in asymptomatic individuals.

Sleep system degradation plays a central role in early breakdown. After forty, sleep quality often deteriorates subtly. Deep sleep shortens. REM cycles fragment. Circadian timing shifts. AI detects these changes and correlates them with daytime performance, inflammation, and metabolic stability. Sleep degradation accelerates aging across all systems. AI does not treat sleep as an isolated issue but as a central regulator of system integrity. What makes AI indispensable is its ability to integrate these signals simultaneously. Humans and traditional diagnostics evaluate systems separately. AI evaluates coordination. It identifies when multiple systems are degrading together, which dramatically increases risk. This convergence of breakdown signals is the true marker of accelerated aging. Recognizing it early allows for intervention before symptoms force drastic action.

AI also distinguishes between temporary stress responses and chronic decline. A difficult week may disrupt sleep and energy temporarily. AI looks for persistence. When disruptions repeat and compound, AI flags them as structural rather than situational. This distinction prevents overreaction while ensuring early action when needed.

Importantly, AI reframes symptoms as outcomes rather than causes. Fatigue, stiffness, brain fog, and mood changes are downstream effects. AI focuses upstream on system interactions. This upstream perspective enables prevention rather than symptom management. After forty, this shift becomes essential for preserving long-term health.

Understanding early system breakdown transforms how aging is approached. Instead of waiting for decline to announce itself, AI provides early visibility into where the body is struggling quietly. This awareness creates opportunity. The earlier breakdown is detected, the easier it is to reverse. The remainder of this book builds upon this principle, translating detection into stabilization and protection strategies.

Before the Pain Arrived

Ethan was forty-eight and considered himself resilient. He worked long hours, exercised inconsistently, and relied on weekends to recover. He felt tired more often than he used to, but nothing hurt. His joints worked fine. His mind was sharp enough. When friends complained about aging, he dismissed it. Aging, he believed, was something you felt when it arrived.

After enrolling in a workplace wellness program that used AI-based health analytics, Ethan agreed to track his data for six months. He expected little insight. What he received was unsettling clarity. The AI revealed that his recovery efficiency had been declining steadily. His heart rate variability failed to rebound after stress. His sleep showed fragmented deep cycles. His metabolic responses were unstable under workload pressure. None of this had produced pain yet, but the system flagged coordinated breakdown across multiple systems.

The AI showed Ethan something he had never considered: he was functioning through compensation. His body was working harder to maintain normal output. This explained why weekends no longer restored him fully. The breakdown was not dramatic, but it was persistent. With guidance informed by the data, Ethan made strategic changes. He redistributed stress rather than eliminating it. He adjusted work intensity, introduced structured recovery, and prioritized sleep consistency. He added strength training to support musculoskeletal stability. Over time, the AI tracked improvement. Recovery curves shortened. Sleep stabilized. Metabolic variability decreased.

Six months later, Ethan felt better than he had in years. What struck him most was that improvement came before pain ever appeared. Without AI, he would have continued until symptoms forced intervention. Instead, he corrected course early, when change was manageable.

Ethan realized that aging does not arrive suddenly. It accumulates quietly. Artificial intelligence had given him a warning before the cost became unavoidable. That warning changed the trajectory of his health long before decline could define it.

Chapter 4

How AI Translates Data Into Early Intervention Instead of Late Treatment

Detecting early aging signals is only valuable if those signals lead to timely action. Traditional healthcare excels at treatment but struggles with intervention because it waits for confirmation of disease. Artificial intelligence reverses this sequence. Instead of asking what is wrong, AI asks what is changing and whether that change is sustainable. After forty, this distinction becomes critical. The difference between early intervention and late treatment is often the difference between preservation and irreversible loss.

Intervention begins with interpretation. Raw data alone does not create clarity. Blood markers, wearable metrics, sleep scores, and activity logs can overwhelm rather than inform. AI converts complexity into meaning by contextualizing each signal within the larger system. It does not isolate a poor night of sleep or a stressful week. It identifies patterns that persist, compound, and interact. This ability to interpret persistence is what allows AI to recommend intervention before damage accumulates. One of the most important shifts AI introduces is timing. In conventional medicine, timing is reactive. Intervention occurs after symptoms cross a threshold. AI introduces predictive timing. It recognizes when trends indicate future instability and recommends action while the body still responds easily. After forty, biological systems retain adaptability, but only if stressors are addressed early. Delayed intervention narrows options and increases required intensity. AI preserves optionality by acting early.

AI-driven intervention is also proportional. Not every signal requires drastic change. AI evaluates severity, velocity, and convergence. A mild decline in one system may require observation rather than action. A moderate decline across multiple systems may require targeted adjustment. A rapid decline in a single critical system may require immediate correction. This proportionality prevents both neglect and overreaction, which are common failures in self-directed health efforts.

Sleep is often the first domain where AI-guided intervention occurs. Because sleep regulates nearly every aging pathway, small improvements yield large returns. AI identifies whether intervention should focus on timing, duration, depth, or consistency. Rather than generic advice, AI recommends specific adjustments based on observed impact. This precision increases compliance and effectiveness. Metabolic intervention follows a similar pattern. AI does not prescribe universal diets. It identifies when glucose variability, energy instability, or insulin response patterns indicate early metabolic stress. Intervention may involve meal timing, macronutrient distribution, or recovery support rather than restriction. This personalized approach preserves metabolic flexibility without triggering unnecessary stress.

Stress regulation is another key intervention domain. AI detects when stress exposure exceeds recovery capacity. It distinguishes between acute stress, which can be adaptive, and chronic stress, which accelerates aging. Intervention may involve workload redistribution, recovery scheduling, or autonomic regulation practices. The goal is not stress elimination but stress balance. AI provides objective feedback that prevents denial and guesswork.

Musculoskeletal intervention is guided by movement data rather than appearance or weight. AI identifies early strength loss, asymmetry, and compensation patterns. Intervention focuses on preservation rather than rehabilitation. This prevents injury and maintains functional independence. After forty, preserving muscle and joint integrity is one of the most powerful longevity strategies available.

Cardiovascular intervention benefits greatly from AI because early vascular aging is rarely symptomatic. AI detects reduced variability, delayed recovery, and autonomic imbalance.

Intervention focuses on improving adaptability rather than simply lowering numbers. This approach preserves cardiovascular resilience rather than masking decline.

Importantly, AI-driven intervention is iterative. It does not assume initial recommendations are perfect. It monitors response and adjusts continuously. If a change improves one system but stresses another, AI detects the trade-off. This feedback loop prevents well-intentioned interventions from accelerating aging elsewhere. Longevity after forty requires balance, not intensity.

AI also helps prioritize intervention by identifying leverage points. Some changes yield disproportionate benefits. Improving sleep consistency may stabilize metabolism, inflammation, and cognition simultaneously. Preserving muscle may improve glucose regulation, bone health, and cardiovascular function. AI identifies these leverage points by modeling system interactions.

This approach transforms aging management from trial-and-error into guided adaptation. Individuals no longer guess whether a change is helping. They see evidence over time. This reduces frustration and increases adherence. After forty, consistency matters more than novelty. AI reinforces consistency by showing progress objectively. Early intervention also reduces psychological burden. When people wait for symptoms, fear often accompanies action. Early intervention feels proactive rather than reactive. It preserves a sense of control. AI provides reassurance by distinguishing normal fluctuation from meaningful decline. This clarity supports long-term engagement.

By translating data into timely, proportional, and personalized intervention, AI changes the trajectory of aging. Instead of managing decline, individuals manage direction. The remainder of this book builds upon this foundation, expanding into specific systems and long-term optimization strategies that preserve strength, clarity, and independence.

The Adjustment Window

Lena was forty-five when she began tracking her health with an AI-guided platform. She felt generally well but noticed that her energy dipped unpredictably. Some days she felt strong and focused. Other days she felt inexplicably drained. Her doctor saw no issues. Blood work looked fine. The inconsistency bothered her more than any specific symptom.

After several months of data collection, the AI identified a pattern Lena had never considered. Her sleep timing varied significantly, even when total sleep hours were adequate. This inconsistency disrupted her metabolic regulation and amplified stress responses. The AI flagged this as an early intervention window. The system showed that her body still adapted well when sleep stabilized, but adaptation was slowing.

Rather than suggesting sweeping lifestyle changes, the AI recommended a narrow adjustment: consistent sleep and wake times within a forty-five-minute window. Lena doubted such a small change would matter, but she committed to it. Over the next eight weeks, the AI tracked improvements in energy stability, stress recovery, and cognitive consistency.

Encouraged, Lena addressed the next flagged pattern. Her movement data revealed early muscle imbalance and declining recovery after high-intensity exercise. The AI recommended modest resistance training and adjusted recovery scheduling. Again, the change was small but targeted. Within months, Lena felt more stable physically and mentally than she had in years.

What struck Lena most was timing. None of these interventions would have occurred if she had waited for symptoms. The window was subtle and temporary. AI had identified it precisely when action required minimal effort and produced maximal benefit.

By forty-seven, Lena's metrics reflected improved resilience across multiple systems. She did not feel younger in a dramatic way. She felt steadier, clearer, and more capable. The adjustment window had closed behind her, but she had passed through it intentionally rather than stumbling into decline.

Lena learned that aging is not just about what you do, but when you do it. Artificial intelligence had not changed her life overnight. It had helped her act at the right moment. And that timing made all the difference.

Chapter 5

How AI Builds Personalized Longevity Models Instead of Generic Health Advice

One of the greatest failures of traditional health guidance after forty is generalization. Advice is delivered in averages, recommendations are standardized, and risk is assessed based on population norms. Yet aging does not occur in populations. It occurs in individuals. Artificial intelligence fundamentally changes longevity science by abandoning generic advice and replacing it with personalized aging models that adapt continuously as the body changes.

After forty, individuality matters more than ever. Genetics begin to express differently. Hormonal shifts alter how stress, nutrition, and exercise are tolerated. Life context diverges widely. Two people with identical lab results may respond in opposite ways to the same intervention. AI accounts for this by building models that learn from your unique data rather than forcing you into statistical categories.

A personalized longevity model begins with baseline mapping. AI integrates historical data such as blood markers, movement patterns, sleep architecture, stress responses, recovery curves, and lifestyle inputs. Rather than comparing you to others, AI compares you to yourself over time. This self-referential approach reveals whether change is occurring and in which direction. After forty, direction is more important than position.

These models are dynamic, not static. Traditional health plans assume stability. AI assumes change. Every intervention becomes an experiment. The model observes how your body responds and adjusts recommendations accordingly. If an intervention improves one system but stresses another, AI detects the imbalance. This prevents unintended consequences, which are common when following generalized advice.

Personalized models also account for trade-offs. Longevity is not about maximizing every metric simultaneously. Improving endurance at the expense of recovery may accelerate aging. Aggressive calorie restriction may impair hormonal balance. AI evaluates these trade-offs in real time, prioritizing long-term system stability over short-term performance gains.

Stress tolerance is a critical personalization variable after forty. Some individuals adapt well to high cognitive load but poorly to physical stress. Others recover quickly from exercise but slowly from emotional strain. AI identifies these patterns and tailors interventions accordingly. This prevents burnout and overtraining, both of which accelerate aging silently. Sleep personalization is equally important. Optimal sleep duration, timing, and structure vary by individual. AI identifies what restores your nervous system most effectively rather than prescribing universal sleep rules. This precision improves adherence and outcomes.

Nutritional personalization extends beyond macros. AI evaluates timing, variability, and metabolic response. It identifies whether your system benefits from consistency or flexibility, from earlier or later meals, from higher or lower carbohydrate exposure. After forty, metabolic personalization is one of the most powerful longevity tools available.

Movement personalization preserves musculoskeletal health. AI identifies which movements improve resilience and which create compensation. It tailors intensity, volume, and recovery to your adaptive capacity. This prevents injury while preserving strength and independence.

The most important feature of AI longevity models is feedback. Progress is measured objectively rather than emotionally. This reduces frustration and increases consistency. When individuals see measurable improvement, motivation becomes sustainable.

AI also personalizes risk prediction. It identifies which systems are most vulnerable and which are most resilient. This prioritization prevents wasted effort and focuses energy where it matters most. After forty, efficiency matters.

Over time, the model becomes increasingly accurate. Each data point refines predictions. Each response improves personalization. Longevity becomes a guided process rather than guesswork. This transforms aging from something that happens to you into something you actively manage.

Personalized longevity models also evolve with life changes. Stress increases, routines shift, priorities change. AI adapts accordingly. This flexibility is essential for long-term success.

By replacing generic advice with adaptive personalization, AI provides a sustainable framework for aging well after forty. The remainder of this book builds on this foundation, exploring how these models are maintained and refined across decades.

The Plan That Finally Fit

Michael had tried everything by the time he turned fifty. Diets, workout programs, supplements, sleep hacks. Some worked briefly. Most failed quietly. The problem was never motivation.

It was mismatch. Every plan felt slightly wrong, like wearing shoes that almost fit.

At his wife's urging, Michael enrolled in an AI-guided longevity program. The system collected data patiently, without judgment. It analyzed his sleep, movement, stress, and metabolic responses. Instead of telling him what he should do, it showed him how his body actually responded.

The first revelation was stress tolerance. Michael handled physical strain well but struggled with cognitive overload. Late-night work destroyed his sleep quality, which in turn destabilized his energy and mood. No plan had ever accounted for this. The AI did.

The second revelation was recovery. Michael did not need harder workouts. He needed better timing and longer recovery windows. When intensity aligned with his recovery capacity, strength improved without fatigue.

Nutrition was adjusted gently. No extreme restrictions. Just timing and composition changes that stabilized his metabolism. The AI tracked response carefully. When something worked, it stayed. When it didn't, it changed.

Within months, Michael stopped feeling like he was fighting his body. The plan fit because it was his. Not an average. Not a trend. A model built around his biology.

At fifty-two, Michael felt more capable than he had at forty-five. Not because he worked harder, but because the system worked smarter. AI had not given him discipline. It had given him alignment.

For the first time, aging felt manageable. Personal. Intentional. The plan finally fit, and with it came consistency he could sustain for decades.

Chapter 6

How AI Stabilizes Aging Trajectories Instead of Chasing Short-Term Fixes

One of the most overlooked realities of aging after forty is that decline rarely comes from a single bad habit or isolated event. It comes from instability. Fluctuating sleep, inconsistent recovery, repeated metabolic stress, and irregular workload patterns gradually erode resilience. Many people attempt to counter this erosion with short-term fixes—new supplements, aggressive training programs, restrictive diets, or intermittent "resets." Artificial intelligence reveals why these approaches often fail. Longevity is not built by intensity. It is built by stability, and AI is uniquely equipped to measure and maintain it.

Stability does not mean stagnation. It means predictable recovery, reliable energy, consistent adaptation, and sustainable stress tolerance. AI evaluates stability by tracking variance rather than averages. A person with occasional excellent days but frequent crashes is aging faster than someone with steady, moderate performance. After forty, the nervous system, metabolic system, and musculoskeletal system all respond poorly to volatility. AI identifies volatility patterns long before they become symptoms.

One of the first ways AI stabilizes aging trajectories is by identifying hidden oscillations. These oscillations may appear as cycles of productivity followed by exhaustion, intense exercise followed by prolonged soreness, or disciplined routines followed by abandonment. AI does not interpret these as motivation problems. It interprets them as system overload. When stress repeatedly exceeds recovery capacity, the body compensates temporarily but destabilizes long-term. AI detects this imbalance and recommends recalibration rather than escalation.

Sleep stability is a foundational lever. AI tracks not only sleep duration but timing consistency, stage distribution, and recovery impact. It identifies when irregular sleep schedules destabilize circadian rhythms, hormonal signaling, and autonomic balance. Stabilizing sleep often produces cascading improvements across metabolism, cognition, mood, and immune function. AI prioritizes sleep consistency because it multiplies benefits without adding stress.

Metabolic stability is another critical domain. After forty, many people experience glucose volatility even with normal lab results. AI identifies patterns of energy spikes and crashes, post-meal instability, and overnight metabolic stress. Rather than recommending extreme dietary changes, AI focuses on stabilizing inputs. Consistent timing, balanced composition, and appropriate recovery reduce metabolic noise. Stability preserves flexibility without triggering compensatory stress responses.

Stress exposure must also be stabilized, not eliminated. AI distinguishes between productive stress that enhances adaptation and chronic stress that erodes resilience. It evaluates workload distribution, emotional strain, and recovery adequacy. Stabilization may involve redistributing effort, introducing predictable recovery periods, or reducing cumulative overload. This approach preserves capacity while preventing burnout, a common accelerator of aging after forty.

Movement stability protects the musculoskeletal system. AI identifies when training intensity fluctuates excessively or when recovery is insufficient. It detects compensation patterns that arise from fatigue rather than injury. Stabilizing movement volume and recovery preserves muscle, joints, and connective tissue. This prevents the injury-repair cycle that accelerates aging and reduces confidence in physical capability.

Cognitive stability is equally important. AI tracks focus consistency, reaction time variability, and stress-related cognitive decline. Mental performance that fluctuates widely indicates nervous system strain. Stabilizing cognitive demands through pacing, sleep alignment, and recovery preserves clarity and emotional regulation. After forty, cognitive stability contributes directly to perceived quality of life.

What differentiates AI-guided stabilization from traditional advice is feedback precision. AI measures whether stability is improving. It detects when variance decreases, recovery curves smooth out, and adaptation becomes reliable. This feedback reinforces behaviors that work and discourages those that destabilize. Over time, stability becomes self-sustaining because the body experiences fewer crashes.

AI also prevents the false sense of progress that comes from short-term gains. Rapid improvements followed by regression often indicate overreach. AI flags these patterns early, allowing course correction before damage accumulates. Longevity is not about peaks. It is about maintaining capacity year after year.

Stabilization does not reduce ambition. It refines it. AI helps individuals pursue goals within adaptive limits. Strength improves without injury. Energy increases without burnout. Cognitive performance sharpens without exhaustion. This balanced progression is the hallmark of intelligent aging.

By stabilizing aging trajectories, AI shifts focus from reacting to problems toward maintaining equilibrium. This equilibrium preserves optionality. When systems are stable, adaptation remains possible. When systems are volatile, adaptation narrows. After forty, preserving adaptability is the ultimate longevity strategy.

The remainder of this book builds upon stabilization by exploring how AI maintains resilience over decades. Stability is not static. It evolves with life stages, stressors, and priorities. AI ensures that evolution remains aligned with long-term health rather than short-term survival.

The End of the Crash Cycle

Rachel was forty-nine and deeply familiar with extremes. She worked intensely, exercised hard when motivated, and rested only when exhaustion forced her to stop. Her life moved in cycles of productivity and collapse. During high-output periods, she felt unstoppable. During crashes, she felt older than her years. Doctors found nothing wrong. Friends praised her drive. Yet the pattern was wearing her down.

When Rachel began using an AI-guided longevity system, she expected advice to push harder or recover faster. Instead, the AI revealed the core issue: instability. Her sleep varied wildly. Her workouts oscillated between intense and nonexistent. Her workload spiked unpredictably. The AI showed how each oscillation compounded stress across systems. Rather than recommending more effort, the AI recommended smoothing the curve. Rachel resisted at first. Consistency felt boring. Yet she agreed to try. She stabilized sleep timing. She adopted moderate, regular movement instead of extreme workouts. She redistributed work intensity across the week. None of the changes felt impressive.

Over time, the AI tracked declining variance. Energy stabilized. Recovery improved. Cognitive clarity became reliable rather than occasional. Rachel noticed something unexpected: she stopped crashing. Productivity became sustainable. Strength increased without soreness. Motivation no longer depended on adrenaline.

At fifty-one, Rachel reflected on the shift. She had not lowered her standards. She had aligned them with her biology. Stability had not limited her. It had freed her.

For the first time in years, Rachel trusted her body to show up consistently. Artificial intelligence had not given her discipline. It had shown her the cost of volatility and the power of balance. The crash cycle ended not with a breakthrough, but with stability.

Chapter 7

How AI Preserves Resilience and Adaptability as the Body Ages

Stability protects the body from decline, but resilience determines how long that protection lasts. After forty, the true measure of longevity is not how stable life appears during calm periods, but how well the body adapts when stress, disruption, illness, or change inevitably occurs. Aging accelerates when adaptability declines. Artificial intelligence plays a critical role in longevity because it continuously evaluates not only how stable your systems are, but how resilient they remain under pressure.

Resilience is the ability to absorb stress and return to baseline without loss of function. Adaptability is the capacity to adjust to new demands without excessive cost. These qualities peak earlier in life and gradually decline unless actively preserved. AI detects early loss of resilience long before it is felt subjectively. It measures how systems respond to disruption, not just how they perform under ideal conditions.

One of the first indicators of declining resilience after forty is delayed recovery. Stress that once resolved overnight now lingers for days. Illness recovery takes longer. Emotional stress produces prolonged fatigue or cognitive fog. AI tracks recovery curves following physical, metabolic, emotional, and cognitive stressors. It identifies when recovery is incomplete or progressively slower. This change often precedes noticeable decline by years.

Another marker of reduced adaptability is rigidity. Rigid systems respond poorly to variation. Small schedule changes disrupt sleep. Minor dietary shifts destabilize energy. Unexpected workloads trigger disproportionate fatigue. AI identifies rigidity by analyzing response variability. When small inputs produce large disruptions, adaptability is declining. Resilient systems absorb variability without cascading effects.

The nervous system plays a central role in resilience. After forty, autonomic balance often shifts toward chronic sympathetic activation. This state preserves short-term performance but reduces long-term adaptability. AI evaluates autonomic tone through heart rate variability, stress reactivity, and recovery patterns. When sympathetic dominance persists, resilience erodes. AI-guided interventions restore balance before burnout or chronic fatigue emerges.

Metabolic resilience is equally important. A resilient metabolic system handles variation in meals, activity, and sleep without instability. AI detects loss of metabolic resilience through exaggerated glucose responses, energy crashes, and delayed recovery after dietary variation. Preserving metabolic adaptability reduces aging risk across multiple systems.

Musculoskeletal resilience determines independence later in life. AI evaluates how the body responds to load, imbalance, and fatigue. It identifies whether strength and coordination recover fully or whether micro-injuries accumulate. Loss of physical resilience increases injury risk and accelerates functional decline. Early detection allows for targeted reinforcement rather than rehabilitation.

Cognitive resilience protects clarity, emotional regulation, and decision-making. AI tracks how cognition responds to stress, fatigue, and disruption. Increased variability in focus or emotional control signals declining adaptability. These changes are often mistaken for personality or motivation issues. AI reframes them as physiological signals that can be corrected.

Sleep resilience is another overlooked domain. A resilient sleep system recovers quickly after disruption. AI detects when sleep debt accumulates or when circadian rhythms fail to realign. Loss of sleep resilience accelerates aging across all systems. AI-guided stabilization restores sleep adaptability without rigid rules. What makes AI uniquely effective is its ability to test resilience safely. Life inevitably introduces stressors. AI observes how the body responds and learns which systems are vulnerable. It then recommends reinforcement before vulnerability becomes failure. This approach turns stress into information rather than damage.

Resilience preservation requires variation within limits. Total rigidity reduces adaptability. Total chaos accelerates decline. AI identifies the optimal zone where systems are challenged enough to remain flexible but not overwhelmed. This balance shifts with age, stress exposure, and life context. AI adapts continuously to maintain it.

Another key function of AI is preventing resilience debt. When stress accumulates faster than recovery, resilience is borrowed from the future. AI identifies this pattern early, allowing correction before debt becomes permanent loss. After forty, avoiding resilience debt is one of the most important longevity strategies.

Preserving adaptability also preserves independence. Individuals who maintain resilience recover faster from illness, injury, and life disruption. They retain confidence in their bodies and minds. This confidence reinforces engagement, movement, and curiosity, which further support longevity. AI supports this positive feedback loop by making resilience visible and measurable. By focusing on adaptability rather than perfection, AI reframes aging as an ongoing learning process. The goal is not to avoid stress, but to respond to it intelligently. The remainder of this book continues this trajectory, showing how resilience and adaptability compound across decades when guided by intelligent feedback.

Bending Without Breaking

Thomas was fifty-three when he realized his body had become fragile in ways he could not explain. He was not weak, sick, or inactive. Yet small disruptions affected him disproportionately. A late night ruined the next two days. A minor illness lingered. Unexpected stress left him drained longer than before. He felt as though his margin for error had disappeared.

When Thomas began using an AI-guided longevity platform, the system focused not on what he did daily, but on how he responded when things went wrong. The data revealed delayed recovery across multiple systems. His heart rate variability took days to rebound. His sleep failed to normalize after disruption. His energy fluctuated wildly after stress.

The AI explained the issue clearly: his systems were stable under routine conditions but brittle under variation. He had lost adaptability. This insight changed everything. Instead of chasing performance, Thomas focused on resilience. Interventions were subtle. Recovery periods became intentional rather than accidental. Stress exposure was distributed rather than concentrated. Sleep consistency was prioritized without rigidity. Movement emphasized coordination and recovery over intensity. The AI monitored response carefully.

Over months, recovery curves improved. Disruptions no longer cascaded. Thomas noticed that unexpected challenges no longer derailed him. He bent instead of breaking. Confidence returned not because life became easier, but because his body adapted again.

At fifty-five, Thomas reflected on the shift. Aging had not weakened him suddenly. It had narrowed his adaptability quietly. Artificial intelligence had revealed that narrowing while it was still reversible.

Thomas no longer feared disruption. He trusted his ability to recover. Resilience had become his new measure of youth, and adaptability his most valuable asset.

Chapter 8

How AI Prevents Chronic Disease by Identifying Risk Long Before Diagnosis

Chronic disease rarely begins where it is diagnosed. It begins years earlier as subtle dysfunction across multiple systems that remain below clinical thresholds. After forty, the greatest health threat is not acute illness but the slow accumulation of unmanaged risk. Artificial intelligence transforms chronic disease prevention by identifying risk trajectories early, long before symptoms force medical intervention. This shift—from diagnosis to prediction—is one of the most powerful longevity advantages AI offers.

Traditional medicine defines disease using fixed thresholds. Blood pressure becomes hypertension at a specific number. Blood sugar becomes diabetes after crossing a defined line. Cholesterol becomes dangerous only when it exceeds a cutoff. AI rejects this binary framework. It evaluates direction, velocity, and interaction. A value that is technically "normal" but trending steadily upward across years signals far more risk than a temporarily elevated value that stabilizes. AI identifies disease before it has a name. After forty, chronic disease risk often emerges from convergence. Metabolic instability combines with low-grade inflammation. Poor sleep amplifies stress hormones. Muscle loss reduces glucose disposal. Cardiovascular strain increases silently. Each factor alone may seem insignificant. Together, they form a disease pathway. AI detects these convergences by modeling system interactions rather than isolated markers.

Metabolic disease is one of the earliest and most common outcomes of unmanaged aging. AI identifies early insulin resistance through glucose variability, post-meal response patterns, and energy instability. These signals appear years before diabetes develops. Early intervention preserves metabolic flexibility without aggressive restriction, preventing downstream damage to cardiovascular, neurological, and musculoskeletal systems.

Cardiovascular disease follows a similar trajectory. AI detects arterial aging, autonomic imbalance, and recovery impairment long before heart disease is diagnosed. By identifying these trends early, AI enables intervention that maintains vascular resilience rather than reacting to structural damage. This approach reduces the likelihood of major events rather than managing them after occurrence.

Neurodegenerative risk also develops quietly. Cognitive decline often begins with inconsistency rather than loss. AI tracks subtle changes in focus stability, reaction time variability, sleep-brain synchronization, and stress response. These early signals allow for intervention that preserves cognitive reserve rather than compensating for loss later in life.

Musculoskeletal degeneration contributes indirectly to chronic disease by reducing movement capacity. AI detects early weakness, imbalance, and recovery impairment that precede joint degeneration and frailty. Preventing physical decline preserves independence and reduces secondary disease risk associated with inactivity.

Inflammation is a unifying driver of chronic disease. AI evaluates inflammatory burden not only through biomarkers but through physiological response patterns. It identifies when inflammation becomes chronic rather than situational. Early correction prevents cellular damage that accelerates aging and disease development.

AI also identifies behavioral risk accumulation. Inconsistent routines, chronic stress exposure, and recovery deficits compound over time. AI recognizes these patterns objectively, removing emotional bias. This clarity allows for targeted correction before habits solidify into disease pathways.

One of AI's greatest strengths is risk compression. Rather than eliminating risk entirely, AI reduces the duration and intensity of high-risk states. This compression dramatically lowers lifetime disease burden. Living longer is less important than living longer without disease. AI shifts the curve toward extended healthspan rather than prolonged decline.

AI-guided prevention also reduces healthcare burden. Early intervention requires fewer resources and produces better outcomes. Individuals experience fewer crises, less invasive treatment, and greater autonomy. After forty, autonomy becomes a defining feature of quality of life.

Importantly, AI does not promise disease immunity. It provides visibility and choice. By understanding risk early, individuals decide how aggressively to intervene. This empowerment transforms prevention from fear-driven compliance into informed action.

Preventing chronic disease also protects psychological well-being. Living under constant uncertainty accelerates stress and aging. AI replaces uncertainty with information. When risk is understood and managed, anxiety decreases and engagement increases.

By identifying disease risk long before diagnosis, AI shifts the narrative of aging from inevitability to agency. The goal is not to avoid aging, but to avoid preventable decline. This proactive approach defines modern longevity science. The remainder of this book builds toward integration—how these preventive strategies combine into a cohesive aging blueprint that remains effective across decades.

The Diagnosis That Never Came

Elaine was fifty-one when her mother was diagnosed with type 2 diabetes and heart disease within the same year. The news shook her. Genetics were not on her side. Doctors advised regular checkups and lifestyle awareness, but no immediate action was recommended. Elaine felt trapped between fear and inaction.

At the suggestion of a friend, Elaine enrolled in an AI-driven health monitoring program focused on disease prevention. She expected reassurance. Instead, the system revealed early risk convergence. Her glucose levels were technically normal but increasingly volatile. Her sleep fragmentation elevated inflammatory signals. Her activity patterns showed declining metabolic resilience. No diagnosis applied, but the trajectory was clear.

The AI did not alarm her. It explained. It showed how small, repeated stressors were pushing her systems toward disease. More importantly, it showed how reversible the process still was. Elaine made targeted adjustments. Meal timing stabilized glucose. Sleep consistency reduced inflammation. Strength training improved metabolic flexibility. Stress redistribution improved recovery. None of the changes felt extreme. The AI tracked response continuously.

Over time, risk markers stabilized. Glucose variability decreased. Cardiovascular recovery improved. Inflammatory patterns softened. Elaine's biological trajectory shifted away from disease.

At fifty-four, Elaine reviewed her data with quiet relief. She had not avoided genetics. She had outpaced them. The diagnosis her mother received never came—not because of luck, but because risk had been addressed early.

Elaine learned that disease does not appear suddenly. It forms quietly when signals are ignored. Artificial intelligence had given her time, clarity, and choice. That knowledge changed her future before it was ever threatened.

Chapter 9

How AI Restores and Protects Energy as the Body Ages

Loss of energy is one of the earliest and most misunderstood signs of aging after forty. Many people accept fatigue as inevitable, attributing it to work, stress, or responsibilities rather than biological change. In reality, chronic fatigue is rarely caused by a single factor. It emerges from inefficiency across multiple systems that quietly erode the body's ability to produce, distribute, and recover energy. Artificial intelligence changes how energy loss is understood by identifying the exact sources of inefficiency long before exhaustion becomes normalized.

Energy is not a single resource. It is the product of coordinated metabolic function, mitochondrial efficiency, nervous system balance, hormonal signaling, sleep quality, and recovery capacity. After forty, these systems often remain functional but less synchronized. AI detects this desynchronization by analyzing patterns rather than symptoms. It identifies where energy is being lost, misallocated, or overconsumed.

One of the earliest contributors to declining energy is mitochondrial inefficiency. Mitochondria generate cellular energy, and their performance declines subtly with age. AI detects this decline indirectly through recovery speed, metabolic variability, exercise tolerance, and fatigue patterns. Rather than waiting for clinical markers, AI identifies early inefficiency and supports interventions that restore energy production capacity.

The nervous system plays a central role in perceived energy. Chronic sympathetic activation creates a state of constant alertness that masks fatigue temporarily but accelerates depletion. AI evaluates autonomic balance through heart rate variability, stress reactivity, and recovery curves. It identifies when energy is being borrowed from future capacity rather than generated sustainably. Restoring balance reduces fatigue without stimulants.

Hormonal signaling also affects energy availability. Cortisol dysregulation, insulin instability, and declining anabolic signals reduce efficiency. AI evaluates hormonal influence through patterns of alertness, sleep disruption, stress response, and recovery. Rather than treating hormones directly, AI addresses upstream drivers that restore natural regulation.

Sleep is the primary energy restoration system. After forty, sleep fragmentation often reduces energy even when duration appears adequate. AI analyzes sleep architecture, timing, and recovery impact. It identifies whether energy loss stems from insufficient deep sleep, disrupted REM cycles, or circadian misalignment. Correcting sleep inefficiency restores energy more effectively than increasing sleep duration alone.

Metabolic instability is another major energy drain. Glucose fluctuations, delayed recovery after meals, and inconsistent fueling increase fatigue. AI detects these patterns and recommends stabilization rather than restriction. When metabolism stabilizes, energy becomes predictable and sustainable.

Muscle mass preservation also influences energy. Muscle acts as a metabolic regulator and energy buffer. AI identifies early muscle loss or reduced activation that increases fatigue. Preserving muscle improves energy efficiency across systems.

AI also identifies behavioral energy leaks. Irregular routines, cumulative stress exposure, and poor recovery timing compound fatigue. AI provides objective insight into how daily patterns drain energy over time. This clarity allows for correction before exhaustion becomes chronic.

One of AI's greatest advantages is distinguishing between true energy deficit and perceived fatigue. Some fatigue is neurological rather than metabolic. AI differentiates these states by analyzing performance consistency and recovery patterns. This prevents inappropriate interventions that worsen fatigue.

Energy restoration requires prioritization. AI identifies which changes yield the greatest return. Improving sleep consistency may restore energy across multiple systems simultaneously. Reducing stress volatility may improve mitochondrial efficiency and hormonal balance. AI identifies these leverage points precisely.

Importantly, AI reframes energy as a renewable resource when managed intelligently. After forty, energy must be protected, not exploited. AI supports sustainable output rather than peak performance followed by collapse. This approach preserves vitality across decades.

Protecting energy also protects motivation and engagement. Chronic fatigue reduces movement, curiosity, and social interaction, accelerating aging. Restored energy reverses this cascade. AI supports this positive feedback loop by making progress measurable.

By restoring energy at the systems level, AI prevents fatigue from becoming a defining feature of aging. The goal is not endless stimulation, but reliable vitality that supports work, relationships, and independence. This restoration prepares the foundation for the final chapter, where all systems integrate into a unified aging blueprint.

The Quiet Return of Stamina

Patrick was fifty-two when he realized his world had quietly shrunk. He still worked, exercised occasionally, and maintained responsibilities, but everything required more effort. He planned his days around energy conservation. Afternoons felt heavy. Evenings were often lost to exhaustion. Doctors found no explanation. "It's just age," he was told.

Reluctantly, Patrick began using an AI-based longevity platform focused on energy optimization. The system did not ask how tired he felt. It asked how his body responded to stress, sleep, and recovery. Over weeks, patterns emerged. His sleep was fragmented. His stress response never fully shut off. His workouts drained more energy than they restored. His metabolism fluctuated unpredictably.

The AI explained that Patrick's fatigue was not a lack of effort but a loss of efficiency. His systems were consuming energy faster than they regenerated it. The solution was not more rest or more stimulation. It was synchronization.

Interventions were subtle. Sleep timing stabilized. Workload intensity was redistributed. Strength training replaced excessive cardio. Recovery was treated as a priority rather than an afterthought. The AI tracked response patiently.

Within months, Patrick noticed change. Not dramatic bursts of energy, but steady availability. Afternoons no longer felt impossible. Evenings became usable again. He stopped planning life around exhaustion.

At fifty-four, Patrick reflected on the shift. Energy had not returned all at once. It had reappeared quietly, as efficiency improved. He felt capable again, not because he pushed harder, but because his body worked better.

Patrick realized fatigue had never been inevitable. It had been a signal he didn't understand. Artificial intelligence had translated that signal into action. Stamina returned not as youth, but as sustainability.

Chapter 10

The Smart Aging Blueprint: Integrating AI Into a Lifelong Longevity System

Longevity after forty is not achieved through isolated improvements. It is achieved through integration. Each system discussed throughout this book—metabolic stability, sleep consistency, musculoskeletal preservation, cardiovascular resilience, cognitive clarity, stress regulation, energy efficiency, and disease prevention—does not operate independently. They are interdependent components of a dynamic organism. Artificial intelligence becomes most powerful when it moves beyond identifying and correcting individual weaknesses and begins coordinating the entire system. The Smart Aging Blueprint is not a program. It is a framework for lifelong alignment between biology and behavior, guided continuously by intelligent feedback.

The first principle of the Smart Aging Blueprint is visibility. You cannot manage what you cannot see. After forty, biological changes accelerate quietly. AI creates visibility into trends, trajectories, and convergence. It transforms vague feelings into measurable patterns. This visibility reduces uncertainty and replaces guesswork with data-informed decision-making. Longevity begins with awareness, and AI sustains that awareness over decades.

The second principle is prioritization. Not all risks carry equal weight. AI identifies leverage points—areas where small improvements produce broad system benefits. Sleep consistency may stabilize metabolism, mood, and cardiovascular health simultaneously. Strength preservation may improve metabolic resilience and reduce injury risk. Stress redistribution may restore nervous system balance and improve energy efficiency. The Smart Aging Blueprint focuses effort where it multiplies.

The third principle is proportional intervention. After forty, extreme strategies often create more harm than benefit. AI measures the appropriate intensity of change based on adaptive capacity. When resilience is high, challenges can be introduced safely. When resilience narrows, intervention must emphasize recovery and stabilization. The blueprint adjusts continuously to life circumstances rather than applying static rules.

The fourth principle is stability before optimization. Attempting to maximize performance without stabilizing recovery accelerates aging. AI identifies volatility across systems and smooths fluctuations before pursuing improvement. Stability creates the foundation upon which resilience and adaptation can be built safely. The fifth principle is feedback loops. Every action produces a response. AI measures whether interventions are beneficial or destabilizing. This iterative loop refines the blueprint over time. Instead of committing to rigid plans, individuals adapt intelligently based on objective outcomes. This adaptability ensures sustainability across decades.

The sixth principle is adaptability. Aging changes biological tolerance. What works at forty may not work at fifty. AI models evolve with the individual, recalibrating stress thresholds, recovery needs, and intervention strategies. The blueprint is dynamic, not static. It grows with the body.

The seventh principle is resilience preservation. Stability without resilience creates fragility. AI tests how systems respond to disruption and strengthens weak links proactively. This protects independence and prevents minor setbacks from cascading into decline.

The eighth principle is risk compression. Chronic disease is prevented not by eliminating risk entirely but by reducing the duration and intensity of high-risk states. AI shortens these periods through early detection and correction. Over time, this compression significantly reduces disease burden.

The ninth principle is energy sustainability. Energy must be renewable. AI ensures that output does not exceed recovery capacity. Sustainable energy supports engagement, productivity, and quality of life.

The final principle is long-term alignment. The Smart Aging Blueprint is not about perfection. It is about direction. AI continuously evaluates whether biological age is accelerating or stabilizing. When drift occurs, adjustments are made early. Over years, these small corrections compound into profound protection.

The Smart Aging Blueprint transforms aging into an intelligent partnership between data and discipline. It preserves autonomy while leveraging technology. It does not promise immortality or eliminate uncertainty. It offers clarity, adaptability, and informed action.

After forty, the greatest asset is not youth but agency. Artificial intelligence extends agency by revealing what would otherwise remain hidden. The blueprint is a commitment to visibility, stability, resilience, and sustainability across the second half of life.

As you move beyond this book, the blueprint becomes your operating system. It evolves as new tools emerge and new life stages unfold. Aging no longer happens passively. It becomes something you guide intentionally.

The Decade That Changed Direction

At forty-one, Marcus felt healthy but restless. He watched older colleagues struggle with health crises and wondered quietly when his own turn would come. By forty-five, fatigue and stress had begun to accumulate. Nothing dramatic, just subtle erosion. He began using an AI-guided longevity platform after a routine checkup revealed nothing but reassurance.

The system mapped his baseline patiently. It identified volatility in sleep, minor metabolic instability, declining recovery efficiency, and early cardiovascular rigidity. No diagnosis applied. Yet the convergence was clear.

Instead of reacting to fear, Marcus adopted the Smart Aging Blueprint principles. He focused on visibility first, reviewing trends monthly rather than obsessing daily. He prioritized sleep consistency, which stabilized multiple systems simultaneously. He redistributed stress and strengthened his musculoskeletal foundation. AI feedback refined his approach continuously.

At forty-eight, a period of intense professional demand tested his resilience. Sleep faltered. Stress increased. Instead of collapsing into exhaustion, Marcus relied on data. He reduced load temporarily, increased recovery, and stabilized routines.

Within weeks, systems returned to baseline. By fifty-one, Marcus felt more capable than he had at forty-five. Not because he avoided stress, but because he responded intelligently. Biological age metrics stabilized. Energy remained reliable. Confidence increased.

At fifty-five, Marcus reflected on the decade behind him. The changes had been incremental, almost invisible. Yet direction had shifted. Aging had not accelerated as he feared. It had stabilized under guidance.

The decade that could have marked decline instead marked recalibration. AI had not replaced his effort. It had guided it. The blueprint had not demanded perfection. It demanded attention.

Marcus understood that the future would still include stress, illness, and uncertainty. But he no longer feared silent acceleration. He had a system. He had visibility. He had agency.

And that changed everything.

Epilogue

The Second Half of Life, Redesigned

Aging after forty does not mark decline. It marks awareness. It is the moment when biology becomes less forgiving and more honest. Small decisions carry greater weight. Recovery slows. Resilience narrows if neglected. Yet this phase of life also offers something earlier decades rarely do: clarity. With clarity comes the opportunity to redesign the trajectory of the second half of life deliberately rather than reactively. Artificial intelligence is not the hero of that redesign. It is the instrument that makes clarity measurable.

Throughout this book, you have seen how aging accelerates silently, how biological age differs from chronological age, how system breakdown precedes symptoms, how stability prevents volatility, how resilience preserves adaptability, how disease risk converges quietly, and how energy must be protected as a renewable resource. These insights are not isolated concepts. They are parts of a single transformation: shifting from passive aging to guided aging.

The epilogue is not about new tools. It is about mindset. The most profound shift that AI introduces into longevity is not technological but psychological. It replaces fatalism with feedback. It replaces guessing with measurement. It replaces waiting with adjustment. When you can see trends clearly, fear loses its grip. Aging stops feeling like something happening to you and becomes something you influence.

After forty, the margin for error narrows, but the margin for wisdom widens. The body sends signals earlier. AI helps you interpret them accurately. Instead of dismissing fatigue as "just getting older," you examine recovery efficiency. Instead of accepting stiffness as inevitable, you evaluate musculoskeletal resilience. Instead of fearing family history, you monitor risk convergence. You intervene when intervention is easy, not when it is urgent.

Longevity is not about extreme optimization. It is about compression of decline. The goal is to live as many years as possible in strength, clarity, mobility, and independence, and as few years as possible in frailty, confusion, and limitation. AI supports this compression by identifying risk early and stabilizing systems before collapse. It shortens the duration of vulnerability.

One of the most important lessons in intelligent aging is humility. Biology does not respond to force. It responds to alignment. AI reveals misalignment quickly. If you push beyond recovery capacity, it shows up in variability. If stress accumulates silently, it appears in recovery curves. If sleep erodes slowly, it appears in metabolic instability. These signals are not judgments. They are information.

The second half of life is not about reclaiming youth. It is about protecting function. Youth is characterized by excess adaptability. Mature longevity is characterized by managed adaptability. AI does not attempt to rewind time. It protects coordination. It preserves integration across systems. It allows you to move forward without drifting backward.

The most powerful compounding factor in longevity is consistency. Not perfection, not intensity, but consistency. AI reinforces consistency because it rewards small, repeated improvements with measurable outcomes. When sleep stabilizes, variability decreases. When muscle is preserved, metabolic resilience improves. When stress is redistributed, recovery curves smooth. Seeing progress reinforces behavior. Reinforced behavior becomes habit. Habit becomes trajectory.

The blueprint you have learned is not static. It evolves with you. In your forties, early detection dominates strategy. In your fifties, restoration and recalibration become central. In your sixties and beyond, preservation and independence define priorities. Artificial intelligence adapts across these transitions. It does not impose uniform solutions across decades. It grows alongside you. There will be disruptions.

Illness will occur. Stress will spike. Sleep will falter. The difference now is awareness. You will see deviation sooner. You will respond earlier. Instead of waiting for collapse, you will adjust at drift. That single habit—adjusting at drift—is the defining behavior of intelligent aging.

Technology will evolve. New biomarkers will emerge. Digital twins may simulate your future health. Predictive models will become more precise. But the principles will remain constant. Visibility. Stability. Resilience. Risk compression. Energy sustainability. Integration. These are not trends. They are timeless anchors for longevity.

The future of aging will not belong to those who avoid time. It will belong to those who manage direction. Artificial intelligence offers directional clarity. What you do with that clarity remains a human choice.

The epilogue is not an ending. It is a recalibration point. Aging does not accelerate overnight, and it does not stabilize overnight. It shifts gradually, shaped by accumulated adjustments. You now understand how to make those adjustments deliberately.

The second half of life is not a descent. It is a redesign.

The Long Horizon

When David turned forty, he felt invincible. By forty-five, he felt tired. By fifty, he felt cautious. He had not been diagnosed with anything serious, yet something subtle had changed. He recovered slower. His patience thinned. His energy fluctuated. He blamed work, responsibilities, and time.

At fifty-one, after a colleague suffered a sudden health crisis, David began tracking his health through an AI-guided longevity system. At first, it felt clinical. Numbers, trends, variability graphs. But gradually, a pattern emerged. His systems were not failing. They were drifting.

Sleep inconsistency amplified stress. Stress reduced recovery. Reduced recovery increased metabolic instability. None of it dramatic. All of it cumulative.

David chose to act at drift rather than wait for collapse. He stabilized sleep. He redistributed workload. He preserved muscle. He tracked recovery. The changes were modest, almost boring. Yet the data reflected improvement. Variability narrowed. Recovery accelerated. Energy stabilized.

At fifty-five, he experienced a significant stress event—unexpected job restructuring. In the past, such disruption would have triggered exhaustion and months of instability. This time, he adjusted quickly. He monitored stress load, increased recovery, and protected routines. Within weeks, systems returned to baseline.

By fifty-eight, David felt something unexpected: confidence. Not youthful recklessness, but measured capability. He trusted his body to respond. He trusted his ability to adapt. He no longer feared silent acceleration because he recognized early signals.

At sixty, David stood at a shoreline with his daughter, watching the horizon. He realized something profound. Aging had not been an enemy. It had been a direction. For years, he drifted unconsciously. Then he learned to steer.

The horizon looked different now—not shorter, but clearer. He knew there would be storms. But he also knew he would see them forming.

The second half of his life did not feel smaller. It felt intentional.

And intention, he realized, was the real measure of longevity.

www.ingramcontent.com/pod-product-compliance
Lightning Source LLC
LaVergne TN
LVHW022023200926
848481LV00007B/2503